Nursing During the Outbreak:

Outbreak:

What I Saw, What I Felt, and Why I Chose to Stay.

Sheltee Felton

Nursing During the Outbreak:
What I Saw, What I Felt, and Why I Chose to Stay.
Copyright © 2021 by Sheltee Felton

ISBN (978-163848-922-1)

MTE Publishing
mtepublishing.com

Dedication

I dedicate this book to every person that has felt or feels overwhelmed by the circumstances of life, especially those who are concerned with their health. I pray this book comforts your fears and your apprehensions regarding the healthcare system and those who work within it.

iv

Table of Contents

Introduction

Before I proceed, I must provide an abbreviated history of who I am. My name is Sheltee (Debose) Felton. I was born in Gainesville, Florida and raised in the small town of Hawthorne about 10 miles southeast of Gainesville's city limits. Why is this important? Allow me to explain… a few weeks before social distancing began in Florida, Hawthorne Middle/High School won the Varsity Basketball 1A State Championship Title in both girls (February 28, 2020) and boys (March 6, 2020). Their victory was led by two brothers, Cornelius Ingram and Greg Bowie. This was an epically historic achievement!

In one year, both the boys and the girls became champions for Hawthorne Middle/High School. This monumental feat gave the entire town an overwhelming sense of joy and excitement. Our entire city was proud to be a Hornet especially after almost losing our middle/high school a few years earlier, due to poor academic ratings on the state accountability report.

These state titles were extremely significant for the entire community. Around late March, the seriousness of social distancing began in Florida. The Center for Disease Control (CDC) advised that everyone practice social distancing to prevent the spread of the Coronavirus. During our lifetime, we had never experienced a global pandemic. Furthermore, we did not know very much about the Coronavirus aka COVID-19.

When news of the Coronavirus outbreak hit the media circuit, stories and conspiracy theories surfaced from everywhere! From CNN news anchors to celebrity bloggers, everyone was consumed with COVID-19, and many of us still are. LovelyTi, who is a prominent blogger gave a report that stood out to me because she provided information that the news in China excluded intentionally [seemingly]. Her informant reported that this virus originated at a seafood market in Wuhan China, that sold live exotic animals such as birds, koalas, bats, snakes, genital parts of tigers, raccoons, and beavers. Unfortunately, these exotic animals were infected by the

Coronavirus and it was transmissible to humans when they ate these animals.

The Chinese government censored local media and international communication so this pertinent information would not be released to the world. Fortunately, there were a few whistleblowers [heroes] who did not mind sharing this information and willingly risked their lives [in hopes of saving others], despite government censorship.

Dr. Li Wenliang, a 34-year-old ophthalmologist is one of the named heroes because he informed the world about the outbreak. The Chinese government silenced political officials and their citizens because they did not want the reality of the pandemic to get out to the world because they knew they would be blamed for its detrimental aftermath.

Their government attempted to silence Dr. Li by declaring his statements about Coronavirus were nothing more than fallacious rumors. However, Dr. Li's death, which was caused by the Coronavirus proved otherwise.

The citizens of China were terrified to post anything in mainstream because of the inevitable repercussions.

It was hard for me to believe anything that the Chinese government reported because they initially hid the seriousness and deadly realities of the Coronavirus. Furthermore, if they had the virus under control the people of China would not *still* be in protective gear. The first case of Coronavirus in the U.S. was publicized on January 21, 2020, and the virus was broadcasted by the Chinese government on January 20, 2020. Although, I felt uncertain and humanly afraid, I didn't hang up my cape, meant my scrubs... However, I suited up in my work uniform and protective gear because I realized I was needed, and my heart wouldn't allow me to forsake my calling.

Chapter 1

Life and Death in Our Hands

Universal health precautions were in *fuller* effect! Washing our hands for 20 seconds, coughing/sneezing into the inside of our forearm and elbow, intentionally and almost obsessively not touching our faces, eyes, or nose, keeping at least six feet from each other, and wearing protective gear was mandatory and vital for everyone! Life as we knew it seemingly changed in a matter of minutes. The entire world was fighting a fatally unapologetic disease.

The Coronavirus spread from encountering contaminated surfaces and introducing the contaminate to your face and mouth; encountering an infected person's cough/sneeze droplets, or simply breathing in the air that has been contaminated by an infected person could possibly put an individual at risk. If Coronavirus droplets landed on person's clothes, their hair, or any surface it could live for days and potentially infect multiple people.

1

The spread of COVID-19 moved at the speed of light and was so easily transmissible that fear and chaos was inevitable.

As an ICU nurse, I knew the risk of entering a COVID-19 patient's room, the virus immediately latched onto to my scrubs, my hair, and the parts of my body that weren't covered by protective gowns. My angst was indescribable! I constantly wondered if I safely removed my Personal Protective Equipment (PPE) and if I scrubbed my hands efficiently enough to rid them of the virus before eating lunch, *if I even had a chance to eat.*

After washing my hands, I'd sit down at the nurse's station to look over a patient's chart and then I'd wonder if the computer we utilized was contaminated. It belonged to the hospital, so as a healthcare worker, everyone who works for the hospital is free to use it. I found myself wiping down countertops, nursing stations, computers, writing tools, cabinets, and Pyxis (a machine that stores patient's medications). Anything that was constantly touched by others was wiped frequently with a disinfectant.

After completing my shift, I always wondered if I'd done enough to prevent infecting myself and my family upon returning home. When I'd arrived there, I stopped at my front door and I undressed from head to toe, then I threw my contaminated clothing into the washing machine immediately. Then I would go to bathroom and shower. I did this before spending any time with my family. I was afraid of infecting them and they were equally afraid that they may get infected if they got too close to me! This virus hijacked its way into the homes of every healthcare worker physically and mentally, and its presence was inescapable.

I stopped watching the news to escape it and although social media was an outlet before COVID-19, it now consumed social media as well. I tried taking leisurely strolls to decrease my anxiety, but everyone I saw wore the tell-tell sign of looming death – the masks. From grocery store employees to the White House, masks covered everybody's identity and proved COVID-19 had no respect of who a person was! It seemed to be a never-ending story, but it was more like a nightmare on repeat… COVID-19 Groundhog Day, it hogged and stole our attention day and night!

Working as an ICU nurse, has several challenges and one of the challenges is to make sure we protect ourselves and the safety of others. On March 19th, my coworker was caring for a patient who potentially was exposed to the Coronavirus, but she left the negative pressure room door opened. All doors to negative pressure rooms must remain closed, so the virus can be contained and not spread throughout the Intensive Care Unit. I quickly put on a N95 mask and closed the room door. I had to put on the N95 mask due to the location of the patient, by closing the door it would have put me within the recommended 6 feet of the patient.

Soon after this occurrence, we received a patient in the ICU from the emergency room, who was diagnosed with pneumonia. However, the ICU was not told that this patient was on droplet/airborne precaution when the patient arrived. This is a precaution that hospitals use to inform healthcare workers about the type of pathogen(s) that is presented and the type of personal protective equipment we must use to protect ourselves. As we proceeded to get the patient in bed, we did not know that this patient was on droplet/airborne precautions until after the ER staff left.

During this time, I was unsure if the patient was a COVID-19 patient or only a bacterial/viral pneumonia patient. One of our team members looked at the patient's medical records on the computer and saw that the patient was on special precaution. We were afraid because of the potential exposure of the virus and I overheard someone state they were going to write an incident report on this matter. I later found out that both patients in the scenarios above were negative for COVID-19. Thank God, because we are all humans and mistakes can be made in the medical field, but we all have to be more aware of our surroundings and communicate effectively to keep everyone as safe as possible.

COVID-19 testing results around world seemed to be questionable. It was reported that a nurse who was exposed to a Coronavirus patient test came back negative and she questioned whether her Coronavirus test was accurate or not. Her and several nurses had the symptoms of the Coronavirus (cough, fever, shortness of breath etc.) including the glass-like appearance of pneumonia on a CT scan but all their test returned negative. This raised some concerns regarding possible transmission to families and returning to work and exposing coworkers.

On March 30, 2020, I was assigned to care for a positive COVID-19 patient. The patient's symptoms included shortness of breath, low grade fever (highest 100.8°F.), cough, and diarrhea. The night before, the Pulmonologist was really considering intubation due to the patient's lack of oxygen intake and their laborious breathing.

The patient was on a Bi-Pap machine when I was assigned to him and being treated with Hydroxy chloroquine 400 mg twice a day, a drug that treats malaria

I was told if patients are on a Bi-Pap machine and coughs, the virus has an aerosol effect and can last in the air for up to three hours.

I knew that my patient did not care to be on the Bi-Pap mask, because he asked, "How long will I have to be on this mask?" I responded in a kind and assured tone, "Until your arterial blood gases are corrected, and the Pulmonologist says it's okay to remove it."

About mid-day, I placed my patient on 5 liters of Nasal Cannula with the approval of the Pulmonologist, and my patient was content. His breathing measured between 92 percent -93 percent of oxygen. He was placed on a clear liquid diet for nutrition. Throughout the day I encouraged him to drink to prevent dehydration and told him to follow the medical team's instructions so that he could get back home to his family. They had also caught the virus while traveling but only had mild symptoms. However, I knew his family needed him at home.

A couple of days later, he seemed to be improving, still on the nasal cannula breathing roughly 95 percent -

98 percent of oxygen and approximately a week later he was discharged and returned home.

There were many days I felt exhausted, from adding extra layers of protective gear while I constantly moved around and about in the patient's room. I took their vitals, performed assessments, drew blood, and gave medications (which included breathing treatments). During this time, the hospital limited the amount of people who could enter a COVID-19 positive patient's room. Housekeeping and other hospital staff members couldn't enter the rooms. I felt as though I was housekeeping, environmental services, phlebotomist, respiratory therapist, and a nurse all in one.

Additionally, I translated what the physicians needed to communicate to the patients through a sliding glass door. Some physicians chose not to enter the rooms. Instead, they stood outside the patient's room door and spoke to the patients *and* me from a distance, in fear of contracting the Coronavirus.

We stared death in the face daily, while simultaneously holding life and death in our hands. In all the years I had worked as a medical professional, working during COVID-19 has been unlike anything I have ever experienced… but I can't turn a blind-eye or a deaf-ear to my calling.

Chapter 2

Rona, is that You?

On Sunday April 5, 2020 during a screening prior to my shift, I explained that I had a low-grade fever of 98.9 and a few days before it was 99.1. I also mentioned to the screener that I had a scratchy throat, felt winded at times, and I was congested. The screener recorded my information and I proceeded to clock in to work my shift in the ICU.

Approximately 10 minutes later, I received a phone call from the house supervisor… "Nurse Sheltee, we are sending you home because your symptoms are consistent with those of COVID-19. You must follow-up with Employee Health tomorrow." I called Employee Health around 9 a.m. the following day. I was told to monitor my temperature twice a day and when I returned to work, it was mandatory to complete an official screening before I'd be allowed to work in the ICU.

However, on April 7, 2020, I called my doctor and we had virtual appointment. He recommended that I get tested for COVID-19 for precautionary measures and self-quarantine until my results came back. If my results were negative, then I could return to work but if the results were positive, I'd have to continue to self quarantine for 14 days.

On Wednesday, April 8, 2020 at approximately 9 a.m., I was tested for the Coronavirus in a drive-thru at one of the local high schools. I made the decision to go there to avoid a copayment.

The local school drive-thru was free of charge. The nurse who conducted my COVID-19 test, inserted a small Q-tip like swab deeply into my left nostril until he felt resistance, rotated it for about 5 seconds, removed it, and placed it into a small tube with a green top. Then he jokingly said, "Sorry that I made you tear up, now you know how your patient's feel…think of it as payback." We both laughed. He also informed me that my results would be available in approximately five days. I went home to self-quarantine immediately after testing.

On April 9, 2020 (Day 2 of self-quarantine), I woke up and watched CNN news. I saw there were 14,808 reported deaths and 432,438 total coronavirus cases in the United States. Globally 88,630 deaths were reported and 1,487,870 global coronavirus cases according to John Hopkins University.

Hospitals did not have enough PPE, which included N95 masks, gowns, gloves, and face shields. They were also low on ventilators. Hospitals could not meet the demands of COVID-19 because it spread so rapidly! They ran out of beds to take care of patients and had to set up tents and establish unique medical spaces. I thought of them as Pop-up emergency medical centers. Hospital morgues filled to capacity and had to improvise to provide temporary resting places for the deceased patients. Many hospitals purchased semi-trucks with a freezer to preserve their bodies. Funeral directors and city morgue employees became overwhelmed and some even refused to pick up bodies from the hospitals due to the lack of PPE.

On Easter Sunday, April 12, 2020, I woke up and thanked God as I usually do every morning. Later that morning, I praised and worshiped the mighty name of Jesus and our father, God. I felt His spirit consume my body as chills rushed through all over me, over and again, like a tidal wave. After my heartfelt devotion, I watched my cousin, who is a pastor on virtual broadcast.

His sermon covered the resurrection of Jesus Christ and it vividly illustrated how Jesus rose from the tomb, a tomb that was initially meant for a man named Joseph of Arimathea. Joseph of Arimathea took responsibility for the burial of Jesus and placed Jesus in his tomb. However, on the third day, Jesus rose from the dead.

On this day, Easter Sunday, as we celebrated that Jesus Christ overcame death, we were still being reminded that social distancing was mandatory in order to prevent the spread of the coronavirus. The news revealed that the death toll had increased to 21,000 in the United States.

The following Monday on April 13, 2020, I received my results from BayCare via telephone. I was told that my results were negative at the time of taking my test. I was elated and beyond grateful, I began to thank the Lord above! I clicked over to the other line because I had my mom on hold and gave her the news as well, we rejoiced together. Then I immediately gave my son the good news… he was lying in bed. I had not been able to give or receive any affection during my 14-day self-quarantine. I hugged my son, and I gave him a big kiss on his cheek. I could not wait for my husband to get home from work, I was ready to hug and kiss him as well. Having to quarantine and being physically isolated from my family was heart wrenching!

A new report came in on the news and the death toll had reached 22,116 and a total of 557,663 coronavirus cases in America. Hillsborough County, Florida issued a countywide curfew to inform its residents be home between the hours of 9 p.m. - 5 a.m.; to help prevent the spread of the virus. I happily complied with the city's curfew, I felt safer at home anyway.

Chapter 3

Medical Battlefield Certainties

O n April 20, 2020, was my first day back at work in the ICU after getting a negative result for my COVID-19 test. Our floor was busy, but we didn't have any COVID-19 patients. They all had previous pending COVID-19 test that came back negative the day before. I was assigned three patients initially, which is a rarity in our ICU. Usually, the patient o nurse ratio is 2:1.

As soon as I clocked into work and received shift eport from the overnight nurse, I hit the ground running! was extremely busy making phone calls, receiving phone alls, looking up all three patient's labs, medications, getting Cardiac Cath Lab consents for two of my patients, and filling-in as needed. It was one busy morning. I barely nade time for myself. Towards the end of my shift my ower back was killing me, it was hurting so bad my legs

were aching from the constant running back and forth.
was exhausted!

After working for 12 hours, I was finally able to g
home, eat, and rest. The next day, I did it all over agair
When caring for patients, sometimes nurses ofter
sacrifice themselves and work through any pain we ma
feel so we can maximize the healing process of ou
patients and their chances of survival.

The government and CDC appeared to be tryin
to get the pandemic under control and help unemploye
citizens. People all across the U.S. were waiting for th
approval of stimulus checks that would grant $1,200 t
single individuals or $2,400 to married couples and $50
per child. The anticipated disbursement date was April 13
2020.

It amazed me how people unified to help on
another during these difficult times. Volunteers hande
out food to low-income families and unemployed citizens
Local and franchised restaurants prepared and gave fre
food to Hospital staff. People also thought of creativ

ways to celebrate their friends and loved-one's birthday. Artists drew murals of appreciation for frontline-workers on the sidewalks of hospitals, neighborhoods, and businesses.

Large corporations like Starbucks gave free iced coffee, and Krispy Kreme gave free Donuts on Mondays. Several grocery stores opened their doors earlier for the elderly and essential healthcare workers: Publix, Dollar General, Sam's Club, and Winn Dixie were among these selfless businesses.

On the flip side of things, people lost their jobs due to the Coronavirus pandemic. Although, some people had the luxury of working from home and keeping their employment. Schools nationwide transitioned to virtual schooling, and some parents decided to start homeschooling their kids. Sporting events were shut down indefinitely, places of worship were closed, and meat packaging plants were closed down due to staff being infected with the virus. However, they were later reopened by an executive order from the president.

Countless nurses were suspended from work for purchasing personal protective equipment for themselves and their colleagues because the hospitals were low on protective equipment. Some nurses and medical staff were fired because they refused to go into a COVID-19 patient's room because they feared being infected and taking it home to their loved ones. Especially if their loved-one was immunocompromised.

One day after I left work, I stopped at CVS for some medications/vitamins that would minimize the effects of COVID-19 should my family or I ever encounter this virus. As I walked down the medicine aisle, a man in his late 30s to early 40s accompanied by his two young teenagers stopped in their tracks. The father directed his kids to stand on the opposite side of him and away from me as if I were infected. This was when the governor of Florida closed schools because kids were thought to be carriers of the virus. A part of me wanted to say something sarcastically; then I thought maybe he was trying to protect me from them. It amazes me that nurses are perceived as heroes of this country, but we are also viewed as the potentially infected human beings that no one wants to come in close contact with. As soon as we sneeze, cough, or have any inkling of the common cold, people would look at us suspiciously and wonder if our symptoms were caused by the coronavirus. I believe the entire world was on high alert, no one could have the common cold without thinking that it was related to COVID-19.

Home remedies played a major part during this pandemic. People were so afraid of contracting the virus that they were putting Neosporin up their nose, thinking that somehow it would block the virus from being inhaled. People were told to do several things such as: drink hot tea and honey, to gargle their mouths with vinegar, to blow a blow dryer in their face, to eat boogers, to drink vodka, to take street drugs and medications that were used for animals, and to excessively eat bread to drag the virus through the digestive tract to rid themselves of the virus. These measures in fighting the coronavirus mislead people across the world and none of these methods were medically supported.

The entire world was in survival mode, and many people acted as if we were in the middle of an apocalypse! People began hoarding essential items like hand sanitizer, toilet paper, hand soap, disinfectant wipes, bleach, and let's not forget Lysol. The demand for these items caused their price to skyrocket as people feared the country would shut down!

During this pandemic, people with mental health issues, alcohol and drug-related problems, and suicidal tendencies surfaced in the hospitals at an alarming rate. This unfortunate reality was caused by the unavoidable stress from COVID-19. Several individuals felt depressed because of unemployment, social restrictions, and home confinement (people were going stir crazy). However, these measures were necessary in order to help prevent spreading the virus.

The week leading to my mother's birthday which was on March 24th, I desperately wanted to visit her in Hawthorne, Florida. I would have been delighted to see my other family members in Gainesville, Florida as well.

However, due to social distancing and my potential exposure to the Coronavirus, I decided to keep my distance to protect my family, especially my 95-year-old grandmother who was cared for by my mother.

It was hard not being able to travel home to see my family but my love for them outweighed my selfish desire to see them. Eventually, I did a video chat with my mom, sister, and brother via Facebook, it was one of the best days of my life during this pandemic.

Sometimes I wake up in the morning and think, "This is surreal, is there something really going on in our country, and in our world?" Then reality hits, almost instantly... the face masks, the social distancing reminders, the rising number of Coronavirus cases and deaths, the economic impact of the pandemic, and the fact that I care for COVID-19 patients daily doesn't allow me to forget!

Like the rest of the world, I am just ready to get back to what *normal* life was for so many! When we could walk in the grocery stores without a mask, hug each other and shake each other's hands without worrying about contracting the Coronavirus. I want the *normal* that allowed us to gather in large crowds for concerts, theme parks, and vacations with our families and friends.

Sadly, I hoped and wished that things would get back to the way they were… but I knew compliance with the CDC guidelines and diligent efforts to be safe would stop the spread of COVID-19. However, I also understood that our current reality may be our *new normal* for a while.

Chapter 4

COVID-19 is One of 99 Problems

Various events and situations surrounding COVID-19 have been publicized in the media, in the hospitals, and in social life. One situation involving a Navy captain has been stuck in mind since it occurred. The Navy captain was fired for considering the well-being of his sailors before his own. This Navy captain exposed the severity of the coronavirus outbreak on the USS Theodore Roosevelt aircraft carrier, to the media. It was reported that over 100 crew members aboard the ship were infected with the coronavirus. The Navy did not want this information to be publicized.

In the hospitals, many COVID-19 patients died alone because their family members were not permitted to see them! COVID-19 was/is one problem, but it multiplies problems in every facet of our lives and our society.

The mental anguish of COVID-19 seemed to cause several people to be more in tuned with their faith or attempt to continue living "their best lives" while disregarding the danger of COVID-19. One day a pastor in Tampa, FL was arrested because he chose to disregard the social distancing order, which put many lives in danger. Many Pastors and/or Spiritual Leaders conducted virtual services and people attended these services from the comfort of their homes, I was one of them.

The college-aged citizens seemed to have a difficult time "pausing" their social lives. It was reported that several college students were infected due to traveling for spring break. The impulsivity of young adults is often reckless and sometimes fatal.

Nurses are exhausted and distraught, and some have even lost their personal battles with COVID-19 during this pandemic. Nurses have often reused N95 masks and face shields. Although, N95 mask should only be worn once (especially after entering an infected patient's room), since the shortage of PPE, medical staff have had to wear the same mask for the entire shift.

In various states across the US, according to the MSNBC news, some nurses used one N95 mask per week due to the shortage of masks. I was absolutely mortified when I learned of this! God forbid if the person sneezed or coughed while wearing their mask; because the integrity of the mask is now compromised, and the person is now at a greater risk of contracting the Coronavirus.

Some hospitals even had their staff discard the masks in "Mask Only Bins" before leaving in hopes of sterilizing them for reuse. There was no way around leaving the hospital with a mask on or in a person's possession. Medical staff had to leave through their assigned exit door of the hospital. All other doors were locked to monitor everyone who entered and left. Temperature checks were conducted daily for staff and visitors. There were staff assigned to observe their peers to ensure that the N95 mask were preserved, and surgical masks was discarded.

The pharmaceutical world explored a new hope in blocking the Coronavirus, using a drug called Remdesivir. The experimental usage of the drug started in late April of 2020. The drug shortened the recovery period of COVID-19 to approximately 11 days of hospitalization. Remdesivir helps blocks the enzyme that causes the virus to multiply. This drug must be given early on in treatment. It must be given in a hospital setting as an IV infusion for five days.

While frontline workers, pharmaceutical engineers, and the CDC worked diligently to get COVID-19 under control, some businesses reopened, and the stay-at-home sanctions were lifted. On Memorial Day weekend, May 23, 2020, large gatherings were witnessed across the country. People were not social distancing… from the Speedway in North Carolina to the beaches in Florida, from bars in Texas and to the Boardwalk in Ocean City, Maryland, crowds gathered as if COVID-19 was as harmless as losing an eyelash. Thus, Coronavirus cases continued to rise, and death tolls reached staggering numbers that exceeded 100,000 in the United States.

People attempted to justify their selfish negligence by stating their mental well-being was more important than their physical well-being. However, our overall health is what's most important (physical, mental, and spiritual). Some people may ask "Is it worth it?" I say, "It's like holding a gun that is partially loaded… if the gun is aimed at someone, the threat of being shot is just as petrifying as being shot because you don't know if the bullet is in the current chamber or the next one!" We are responsible for ourselves and the choices we make affect ourselves and others.

Within the United States healthcare system and our legal system, the mistreatment of African Americans continues to come to the forefront in a more prevalent manner … cell phone technology/videos seem to be a blessing and a curse. At least, three cell-phone videos have been shown across the world that captured the mistreatment of unarmed African Americans and two of the videos resulted in murder. A Black man named Christian Cooper, was in Central Park bird watching and asked a white woman if she would put her dog on a leash because it was mandatory. The *white* woman did not like the fact that a *Black* man asked her to put *her* dog on a leash. The white woman became enraged and threatened to call the police. She dialed 911 and pretended to be in distress and falsified an alleged pending assault, "There is an African-American man threatening myself and my dog," she pleaded for the 911 dispatcher to send the cops immediately.

Many people believed that the woman deliberately made the fabricated call, in hopes of the police using aggressive force or weapons against the African American man and that this matter would turn out in her favor. Thankfully, this was not the case!

Another incident was the killing of a young educated, unarmed Georgia Black man named Ahmaud Arbery. He was simply jogging and was murdered by two white men. The final racially charged incident of many, was the murder of George Floyd. After Floyd's death was captured on video, the heinous actions and demeanor of the four cops involved caused an immediate frenzy and social unrest. Floyd, as well as bystanders pleaded for his life. He could not breathe because one of the police officers forcefully penned his knee into the back of Floyd's neck, while he was handcuffed and lying prostrate on the ground.

The murder of Breonna Taylor from Louisville, Kentucky was not caught on film. However, she was killed by the police while she slept in the comfort of her own home. Breonna was 26 years old and worked as an EMT. In the middle of the night, the cops raided her home looking for a man who was already in police custody. Later that year, in September, the mother of Breonna received a settlement for a wrongful-death lawsuit, and no one was charged for Breonna's murder.

Although the Coronavirus seemed to initially prompt unity in our society, it also shed light on how divided our country is. I've always thought sickness has a way of allowing us to realize that there is nothing more important than life. Unfortunately for many minorities, especially Black men and women, our lives and humanity are dismissed and deemed invaluable. My hope is that everyone will strive to treat all human beings with dignity and respect.

Chapter 5

In Sickness and in Health

On June 13, 2020 it was reported that within a 24-hour time frame, 2,500 new coronavirus cases would be added to the already alarmingly high number of cases in Florida. Unsurprisingly, we felt every bit of it in the ICU. With one positive COVID-19 patient and at least three rule/out cases we stayed on our feet wearing PPE most of the day. Breaks to use the restroom, eat, drink, or simply catch our breath wasn't an option. It was super busy in the ICU and we were all deliriously exhausted by the end of our shift.

On June 17th, CBS reported over 14,000 new cases in Florida. On Father's Day weekend, June 19th, my family and I decided to get away... so we traveled to Orlando, Florida just to have a change of scenery! We needed an escape (mentally and physically). We had a wonderful time, and we enjoyed each other's company. We wore handmade and surgical masks the entire time except for when we ate. We also had an unexpected visitor come by and she brought a delicious homemade banana cheesecake. We hung out at Disney Springs, ate delicious meals, and did a little shopping. Unfortunately, all good things came to an end and we all returned to our homes.

On Thursday, June 25th, I received a disturbing phone call while at work stating that one of my family members, who was on the trip with the us, tested positive for COVID-19. A few hours later, I received another phone call while at work revealing two additional family members also tested positive for COVID-19. Both calls were devastating, and I couldn't stop myself from sobbing. One of my family members who tested positive was my mom.

My husband decided to go get tested as well because he felt terrible! He had a fever of 102 degrees, body aches, cold sweats, nausea, and loss of appetite, he tested positive. My son and I were tested on Friday, June 26, 2020, with no symptoms, we later received negative results. The day of testing, I read that Florida confirmed lmost 9,000 Coronavirus cases in one day, which was a new record. The Florida Department of Health reported a total of 122,960 Coronavirus cases in the state.

On Saturday, June 27th, I rushed to my mother's house from Tampa to assist her in fighting the Coronavirus. My mom was in pretty bad shape, she had an uncontrolled fever of 102.5. I had to ensure she took Tylenol routinely because she also complained of headaches, body aches, and fatigue.

I reached out to a doctor I knew, because he is a man I highly respect and worked with in the ICU. He advised me to start a regimen of several over-the-counter medications for my mom, the list included Pepcid 20mg twice a day, Zinc 200mg daily, Vitamin C 1000mg every 6 hours, and Melatonin at night to help my mother sleep through her symptoms. I immediately went to the Drug store to purchase all of these items. I prepared a schedule for my mom to take her medications because I knew that I had to leave her because I had to get back to my husband who was also infected with COVID-19.

At times, I felt overwhelmingly depressed as I thought about all of my family members who were fighting COVID-19. I cried as I realized that we could have possibly dodged Rona if we had stayed home instead of traveling to Orlando.

Throughout this process my siblings and I became a team of support and encouragement for our family. We constantly conducted wellbeing checks via phone calls, purchased medications, and we drove back and forth to my mom's house to ensure she was okay. My brother sent daily biblical scriptures to help us remain hopeful and keep our faith strong! James 5:15 and Romans 15:13 became a part of my daily devotion. I'm fortunate to say that all six of my family members who contracted the virus, survived! We thank God that we made it through that season of sickness, and God's grace and mercy allowed us to embrace the wealth we have in health *again*.

Chapter 6

Even Closer to Home

On the early morning of Sunday, June 28th, I felt weakness in my arms. The nasal congestion I had was so bad that I could not sleep. So, I went and got tested for COVID-19, *again*. My test came back negative on Monday, June 29th in Gainesville at an Urgent Care center. The facility gave patients their COVID-19 test results within 20-25 minutes.

Witnessing my mom and husband endure the pain of COVID-19 was heartbreaking. Their temperatures fluctuated from a low-grade fever to a high fever. Therefore, my brother and I had to give them routine fever/pain reducing medications around the clock. My husband lost his appetite, felt nauseated, and experienced slight headaches. Both my mom and husband bodies ached non-stop and they both experienced diarrhea. My mom had a constant cough that at times made her feel short of breath. She could barely talk on the phone without getting winded.

One minute my husband felt awesome and the next minute the virus struck him down again. I encouraged him to keep the faith and believe that God would heal him! Furthermore, I assured him that he would not go through his sickness alone.

My husband received several calls on July 1, 2020… one of his good friends passed away during the morning hours. It was undeniably sad for him, but he knew that his friend had suffered for a while with health conditions unrelated to COVID-19. My husband was unable to attend his long-time friend's funeral because he was still infected with the virus.

It was bothersome that I could not take care of my mom and my husband at the same time because we live in different cities. I thank God that my brother, sister, and nephew were able to assist with helping my mom recover.

This Coronavirus took my loved one's on a roller coaster ride. One minute they felt better and the next minute they felt terribly weak and feverish. At times, my husband's mind would be in a fog, and he could not think straight. His fatigue almost had him in a state of lethargy. My husband wanted to do things for himself, but it took him approximately 30 minutes to do tasks that normally took five minutes [like washing his face and brushing his teeth].

My brother and I constantly encouraged my mom and my husband to eat so they could regain their strength. Their quarantine days were the longest 14 days of my life, but I could only imagine how they felt. They probably could not even imagine the light at the end of the tunnel and their days probably felt endless.

At times I felt feverish and winded but when I took my temperature it was normal, it is crazy how the mind works when we are fearful. My mom's fever finally broke around Thursday, July 2nd, and my husband's fever broke around Saturday night, on the 4th of July. When my husband's fever broke, the shortness of breath slowly started to subside. His health was almost at a 100 percent on Tuesday, July 7th, he felt so good that he made himself a grilled cheese sandwich and he called my brother to share the good news of his recovery.

Throughout my husband's illness, I noticed hypopigmentation areas on his head, circular light patches which had me concerned because I had never seen them before. His skin color returned to normal a few weeks later. My Husband was retested on Friday, July 10th and received his negative results on Monday, July 13th.

My son and I retested to make sure we were *still* negative and because I had mild symptoms. I also wanted to ensure that I was a negative before returning to work because I did not want to infect my coworkers. Our test came back negative, *again*.

At this time, the number of Coronavirus cases and the death toll in Florida increased at an alarming rate. It was reported that 156 people died in a single day in Florida from COVID-19. Florida had 4,782 COVID-19 related eaths. The fatality of the Coronavirus hit so close to ome, that I couldn't help but be grateful! When we stare eath in the face or the possibility thereof at such a close roximity, we put what matters into perspective very uickly… I know I did! All I wanted and needed was to ee my family happy, healthy, and alive!

Chapter 7

Waiting to Inhale and Exhale

Summer vacation for the students all across the United States came to an end. Parents and school district personnel were deciding if traditional school settings would be safe for everyone. Some teachers and students had the option to either go to school or stay at home for virtual classes. Everyone was affected by this decision one way or another.

If students stayed home, they'd miss out on much-needed socializing with their peers. However, if students returned to brick-and-mortar schools they'd risk being exposed to COVID-19. Additionally, several parents felt overwhelmed by the obligation of ensuring that their children were engaged during virtual learning. Teachers had to adjust as well; online teaching and traditional teaching are quite different.

In the month of August some interesting events took place, a 5.1 magnitude earthquake hit in North

Carolina on Sunday, August 9, 2020, a little after 8 o'clock in the morning. The magnitude of the earthquake was felt in parts of South Carolina. Additionally, during this time several news sources revealed a 29-year-old Black man name Jacob Blake, was shot seven times in the back and in the front of his kids by a Wisconsin police officer. He was trying to break up a domestic dispute, the shooting by the policeman left him paralyzed.

Due to this incident, the Milwaukee Bucks decided to boycott their game and a few NBA teams decided to boycott the season. However, the boycott was short lived, because after the NBA spoke with the former President Barack Obama, the team decided to finish up the season.

On Saturday morning, August 29, 2020, the news, and social media were consumed with the devastating death of the "Black Panther" aka Chadwick Boseman. He was a true superhero to the Black community. He passed away at the age of 43 years old due to complications from colon cancer.

It is important to know your family's medical history because if we don't there is no way to know what diseases are hereditary. Screenings for various health conditions or cancers can be performed before the recommended age if the patient has a history of the illness in their family. Early detection is vital for treatment and prevention. Chadwick battled cancer for four years, which would have put him at the age of 39 when he found out he had cancer. Tenaciously he continued to make inspirational movies for the world, especially the Black community. Rest in Power Chadwick, we will love and miss you forever.

As the COVID-19 cases continued to rise in the U.S. and the death toll exceeded 200,000 deaths, Florida's Governor reopened the state at the third phase. Phase 3 allowed gyms, salons, retail stores, theme parks, vacation homes, theaters, and restaurants to reopen at full capacity with no restrictions. One day I walked into a local restaurant to pick up a to-go order and I was utterly appalled! The bar was almost full to capacity and none of the patrons were wearing masks. The recommended social distancing of six feet was ignored, and the scene looked like everything was back to normal… but it wasn't normal. What I saw saddened and worried me because we were still battling a global pandemic.

People felt and believed that due to COVID-19, the focus of medical professionals and primary care physicians was to ensure that patients didn't have COVID-19. Several patients voiced their concerns and they wanted to be assured that they received the best care available to them even if they didn't have the Coronavirus!

Patients also felt that proper hands-on assessments were not being completed because physician could not meet with them face-to-face (which many of them preferred over virtual appointments via Zoom or a teleconference). I understood the patient's concerns and I also understood that physicians had to do everything they could to keep everyone safe from COVID-19… their patients, their staff, and themselves.

On Friday, October 2, 2020 President Trump decided to fly to Walter Reed Hospital after contracting he Coronavirus and feeling fatigued. It was reported that he received a cocktail of Zinc, Aspirin, Famotidine, Vitamin D, and Melatonin. It was also reported that he was given a steroid and an experimental drug [just in case] to help him recover. President Trump refused to wear a mask during this pandemic and even made fun of former Vice President Joseph "Joe" Biden, during the 2020 Presidential debate, for wearing his mask.

President Trump found out he was infected shortly after the debate and I am certain that our country prayed for a speedy recovery on his behalf. Shortly after Trump's recovery, he continued on his campaign trail against former Vice President Joe Biden. One of my main concerns as a nurse during the debate, was getting COVID-19 under control! Medical professionals, nurses, and essential workers have felt the effects of this virus relentlessly. Wearing N95 masks, gowns, gloves, and face shields to protect ourselves, coworkers, family members, and our community continues to be draining and exhausting. We do what we have to do to keep everyone safe.

One day, I spoke with a young male patient who contracted the virus, he stated that he and his mom had contracted COVID-19 from his sister, who had come to visit them from Texas.

This patient took a liking to me, as his nurse, after I shared my personal experiences with him regarding COVID-19. I also told him that he and my son were around the same age. After I explained to the young man how busy I was with all of my COVID-19 patients, I told him that I had to leave. He asked me to hurry back and reluctantly confessed that he felt very lonely after I told him I'd return within an hour.

His statement brought back memories because I could recall how lonely my husband felt when he was battling Covid. Even though I was home taking care of him. The times I was near him, I was armored with my N95 mask, gloves, and goggles. We barely made any physical contact; the only exception was when I had to change his ice packs to keep his temperature regulated. My husband told me he was comforted in knowing that I was nearby, and for entertainment he had Steve Harvey to make him laugh as he binge-watched Family Feud.

I understood what my patient was going through and I asked if he wanted to watch television to keep him occupied. I was extremely saddened for my patient because while he was battling the Coronavirus, he found out that his mom had passed away.

My other COVID-19 patient was an older woman in her 70's, she didn't know how she contracted the virus. She was quite baffled by the ordeal and called it a mystery. Both of my patients survived COVID-19 and were later discharged. My heart leaped for joy every time a patient recovered from COVID-19. These are the realities that made the risk of nursing during the pandemic worth it! Nothing is more precious than life, and it is even more significant when people take the time to care! Patient recovery and happiness made me feel refreshed and I knew eventually I would no longer feel like I was holding my breath…

SHELTEE FELTON

Chapter 8

Hold On, Help is on the Way

It was finally a day of reckoning… November 3, 2020 – the official presidential election day in the United States. Unsurprisingly, 100 million people had already participated in early voting. However, several days after the historic event the American people and the world at large were still anxiously awaiting the results. Several different states including Pennsylvania, Arizona, Georgia, and Nevada were still being counted and recounted.

Finally, on Saturday November 7th around 11:30 in the morning, CNN announced that President Elect Joe Biden had won the 2020 Presidential Election after Pennsylvania completed their ballot counts. Biden had a total of 273 electoral votes and Trump had a total of 213 electoral votes.

The citizen of the United States had spoken, and on January 20, 2021 Joe Biden would be sworn in as the

46th President of the United States and Kamala Harris would be sworn in as the first Black, Indian, and female Vice President. However, remaining true to form, President Trump did not go down without a fight! He filed several lawsuits that challenged the voting process, but none of the lawsuits succeeded.

On November 11, 2020, a new record hit of more than 144,000 new cases of COVID-19 in the U.S. These numbers were calculated from one day and the death rate was equally dismal. Over 65,000 Americans were hospitalized, and Thanksgiving was around the corner. It was predicted that the cases would continue to increase as families gathered for the holidays.

My hope was weakening like most Americans, and COVID-19 seemed as if it was trying to establish permanent residency. Thankfully, pharmaceutical companies were diligently working to produce a vaccine for the Coronavirus, and it would be given to healthcare workers first. I received an email from my employer stating that vaccination companies needed volunteers for linical testing of the COVID-19 vaccine. Others received imilar emails stating that volunteers could be financially ompensated for up to $1,220 if they participated villingly.

Pfizer announced that their vaccine was more than 0 percent effective, and of course the next question was "When will it be available?" As cases continued to rise, numerous hospitals reached and some even surpassed apacity, work life was a daily dose of PTSD. The state of Jtah was depleted of ICU beds due to the influx of COVID cases. The mayor of Chicago issued a Stay-at-Home Advisory Order, which started on November 16, 2020 and was scheduled to last for 30 days, due to the overwhelming death toll of COVID-19.

On Friday, November 13, 2020, President Trump neld a press conference regarding the Coronavirus vaccine. He informed the nation that the vaccine would be available to the American people very soon.

Nurses everywhere were drained mentally, physically, and emotionally. The reality of caring for

COVID-19 patients exceeded exhaustion. The daily obligation of wearing PPE, administering medications, and trying to motivate non-compliant patients to be compliant was almost *too much*.

Imagine feeling suffocated because of a N95 mask while trying to see through a foggy face shield, sweating profusely while wearing a plastic gown and performing physical labor. This was the daily plight while fighting Rona!

Some of our physical labor included constantly dressing in and out of PPE, changing patients and their linen due to uncontrollable diarrhea from the virus, adjusting a severely ill patient in bed to eat so they didn't choke on their food, we had to constantly travel inside a confused patient's room because they'd remove their oxygen which was put in place to help them breath, and having to physically put ventilated and non-ventilated patients in a prone position to help expand their lungs.

Mentally, anxiety set in and we wondered if our PPE kept us protected, because we knew if we were infected there was a high probability that we would also infect our loved ones. Wearing the N-95 mask alone caused anxiety because it caused us to have shortness of breath. Just a simple sore throat sent us into an emotional and mental frenzy because it was one of the symptoms of COVID-19. However, we quickly calmed down because we realized our throats were sore because we'd worn a mask for 12-hours. The filtered air caused our throats to feel dry.

Furthermore, we were emotionally overwhelmed. We experienced sleepless nights and worried about our patients' survival. After caring for any patient, the stress and helplessness we felt if they didn't defeat their illness was depressing. The mental and emotional toll we pay can never be given a monetary value… it is priceless.

The daily report of increasing coronavirus cases and deaths was terrifying. We had to step away from reality, turn off the TV, and log off social media to decrease our stress and angst. Witnessing people struggle to breathe and even worse die from this virus while trying to combat was painful.

At the onset of the pandemic, one morning I sat in my car and contemplated if I would enter the hospital. I did not know what the day would bring but I knew how tiresome and grueling the previous days had been. I listened to Casting Crowns' "Praise You in This Storm" and I bawled my eyes out while praying for God to heal this country and to protect my coworkers and I from this deadly virus. A sudden peace came over me and I felt assured that my heavenly father would protect myself and my coworkers! I knew He heard my cries because I had not contracted COVID-19, although the virus touched me every day!

There have been times that I felt like giving up as a nurse, because I feared the unknown of this virus and I was beyond tired. However, I knew I had to stay the course because the world needed me. It has never been my makeup to just give up, I've always been a fighter no matter how difficult life has been. Undeniably, the

COVID-19 pandemic has been and is one of the hardest periods of my life.

I am and will be eternally grateful for the people who have recognized and shown their appreciation for frontline workers. They brought us food, gave us tokens of love by way of gifts, recognition awards, they detailed our vehicles, and my coworker's mom even made hats and masks for us. I am forever thankful.

One day, while I was waiting in line at the gas station, a stranger offered to pay for my gas, and he would not except "No, thank you" as an answer. I felt uncomfortable accepting this kind and generous act of appreciation because I prefer to be the giver. However, I understood this was his way of saying, "Thank you for everything you've done and continue to do!" To the kind stranger at the gas station, I say, "Thank you," again from the bottom of my heart.

It has been a humbling experience being a nurse during the Pandemic. I'm motivated by helping to save lives and providing comforting care. I realize that I am caring for someone's child, mother, father, sister, brother, aunt, uncle, or friend. Sincerely, I made a professional and personal vow to treat all patients as if they are a member of my family or a friend... and when all else fails, I just tell them to hold on Nurse Sheltee is on the way!

Chapter 9

I Believe in God *and* Science

Thanksgiving is typically a day that many Americans gather with their family and friends to enjoy food, share unforgettable memories and laughter. It is the day that is nationally recognized as a day of gratitude. We openly express our thankfulness for our family, health, and the fact God allowed us to see another day.

Sadly, during Thanksgiving amid the pandemic, many Americans mourned the loss of their loved ones. Thanksgiving (or any other holiday) will never be the same without them, their memories are all they have to hold on to. I said a prayer for these families, I asked God to give them strength to make it through the holidays and I hoped that they were surrounded by people who loved them.

Despite the recommendations to stay home due to the surge in Coronavirus cases, too many Americans traveled to see their love ones for the holidays. Over 2,000 deaths occurred in the United States the day before Thanksgiving. As expected, the number of Coronavirus cases and deaths increased tremendously after the holidays.

On Tuesday, December 2, 2020, CNN announced that the United Kingdom's FDA approved a vaccine, and their citizens would receive the Pfizer COVID-19 vaccination within a week. The U.S. expected to receive the vaccine by the end of December. The Pfizer vaccine required a 2-dose vaccination in order to be effective, and it has an approximate effective rate of 95 percent.

The CDC decided who would receive the vaccine first. People who had a high probability of contracting COVID-19 such as the elderly, people with preexisting morbidities, and healthcare workers were granted first priority.

The second deadliest day during the pandemic was Tuesday, December 1, 2020. Nearly 2,600 people died from COVID-19 complications in the U.S. and it was predicted that approximately 500,000 more Americans could die by March.

On Thursday, December 10, 2020, the U.S. reported 3,100 deaths from the Coronavirus. The FDA met to approve of the Pfizer vaccine for U.S. citizens and thankfully the consensus was a unanimous yes. The vaccine was delivered on Friday December 11, 2020 across America. Some citizens were excited and willing to be vaccinated and others were understandably skeptical.

People wondered if the vaccine was safe, other's felt they had developed immunity because they had been diagnosed previously with COVID-19 and they survived. Then there were some people who believed because they never received a yearly flu shot that the Coronavirus vaccine was unnecessary. Others believed the virus was a hoax…so that meant a vaccine was a part of a conspiracy theory as well.

Two monumental events happened on Monday December 14, 2020, the Electoral College deemed Joe Biden as the next President of the U.S. and the Pfizer

COVID-19 vaccine was scheduled to be administered. The side effects of Pfizer vaccine included: fatigue, fever, chills, muscle pain, redness or swelling at the injection site, and headaches. This vaccine was a series of two injections that were administered three to four weeks apart.

The U.S. ordered approximately 100 million Pfizer vaccines. The first Pfizer vaccine arrived in Kentucky. The first hospital to receive the vaccine was the University of Michigan. Americans were expected to be vaccinated on Monday December 14, 2020. Nearly 300,000 Americans died from this virus prior to the vaccine.

The first person to receive the vaccine lived in New York. The individual was a black female nurse who worked in the ICU at Long Island Jewish Medical Center. This fact is extremely important because I understand the reluctancy and uncertainty that the Black community feels regarding the lack of trust and safety regarding vaccines and our healthcare system. However, I will get the vaccine when it becomes available because I trust in God *and* I believe in science.

Chapter 10

I Am Nurse Sheltee

Being a nurse has its challenges but being considered a hero simply because I care about people is humbling. This pandemic has challenged America to be better in every way possible. If we didn't understand the idea of "life, liberty, and the pursuit of happiness" we surely understand it now!

Too many people died from the Coronavirus and sadly many of them died alone, and it is up to us as a nation to ensure that we live healthy, harmonious, and productive lives. COVID-19 has caused the entire world to feel emotionally, physically, and mentally drained. At times, every fiber of my being told me to quit but my inner warrior wouldn't allow me to walk away. The American people and the world needed committed healthcare workers as much as they needed to breathe! So, I refused to give up. My fellow healthcare workers and I are soldiers on a battlefield, from administrators, physicians, pharmacist and techs, respiratory therapist, patient care techs, case managers, phlebotomist, physical therapist, occupational therapist, Speech therapist, dietary aides and dietitians, cath lab nurses/techs, to radiologist and those who work in environmental services... ALL of us are dedicated to fighting the Coronavirus and we cannot let it defeat us.

Scientists have created a vaccine and we as healthcare professionals are working diligently to keep your loved-ones and ours alive. We are courageous, and we understand that our ability to care for others even when we are afraid is what makes us true heroes.

Therefore, as I end this open letter from the hallways of COVID-19, I ask each of you, the readers to do your part in ensuring that we trounce COVID-19 together. Please continue to wear your mask, wash your hands, and social distance. If you decide to get vaccinated like me, kudos to you! For every person that gets vaccinated we are one step closer to communal immunity.

Finally, I give special thanks to the scientists, healthcare professionals, and essential workers... Your daily sacrifice of service is greatly appreciated!

About the Author

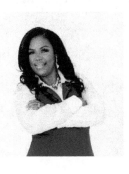

Sheltee (Debose) Felton is more than a nurse. She is a wife, mother, entrepreneur, and *now* a published author! Her life is a testament to the adage, "Life is beautiful, but it becomes perfect when we have people that love and care about us *selflessly*!"

Although, life is quite unpredictable there are people like Sheltee that help everyone to maintain a sense of comfort and balance. Nurses must be heaven-sent because their altruism is divine.

Nurse Sheltee strives to be the caregiver that she would need and want to care for her. She has embraced the golden rule as her mantra, "Treat others the way you want to be treated!" If the world had more people like Sheltee, it wouldn't just be a better place, it would be the best place!

When Nurse Sheltee removes her ~~cape~~, I meant her scrubs… She enjoys quality time with her family, long scenic walks, and relaxing vacations.

CPSIA information can be obtained
at www.ICGtesting.com
Printed in the USA
BVHW082025100521
606946BV00006B/1458

9 781638 489221